# ARE YOU READY TO BE A CAREGIVER?

By

**Sharon Ernst**

# Contents


ARE YOU READY TO BE A CAREGIVER?    5

MENTAL STRESSES    22

PERSONAL HYGIENE    28

FAMILY & FRIENDS INVOLVEMENT    31

MEDICAL PROFESSION    35

MEDICARE HEALTH INSURANCE BILLINGS    39

DEALING WITH GOVERNMENT AGENCIES    42

NURSING HOME/ASSISTED LIVING    46

EPILOGUE    49

# ARE YOU READY TO BE A CAREGIVER?

Making the decision to become a caregiver is a life altering experience, the decision to do so should be given much thought as it will be one of the biggest commitments you will make in your lifetime.

As I began to write about my experiences being a caregiver for my parents for several years I thought it would be a useful tool for those who found themselves in a similar position as I was.  When I spoke with other caregivers I realized that most caregivers had no idea of what they were about to undertake.  There is no guide to tell you what to expect or the depth of involvement that is often required of a caregiver.  This book is intended to help guide you in making the best decision for all parties involved.

My experience as a caregiver was with both parents, one of which had Alzheimer's.   On the following pages I have compiled several questions with my answers to them.  There is no right or wrong answer to the questions. They are all geared to help you understand what lies ahead if you make the decision to become a caregiver for someone.  It is not unusual for responsibilities to increase with the amount of time you are a caregiver.

In that context I hope they will be useful to anyone reading them.  They are meant to make you aware of and think about various circumstances that may or may not occur while you are a caregiver.  I also encourage the reader to add their own questions and answers to fit their situation.

The main point is that you make the best decision for not only yourself but the persons or persons that you could become a caregiver for.

Caregiving should not be gone into blindly, the more information you can gather in advance will aid you in the decisions that you will have to make.

Are You Single?

If you are single and living alone you have your own lifestyle with no one to disagree with you.  You are in command of your life and how you want to live it is your decision.   There is no one that you have to answer to other than yourself.

## Married or in a Relationship?

Is your spouse or mate supportive, taking on this task is very stressful.  It can create problems as to time spent with partner, communicating. and home life.  It becomes difficult to maintain any sense of normalcy, there is never enough time to give to any one person or family.  It is not possible for you to satisfy the needs of all parties involved, causing dissension in one's family.  You try your best to meet all your responsibilities, yet it never is quite enough time to keep everyone happy.


## Do You Have Other Family Members in the Area?

The full load of responsibilities is almost always placed onto one person in the family.  What may have been discussed with other family members pertaining to care and the options available are soon forgotten, once your take on the responsibility.

They most always say they will help, their intentions are well meant, but their actions can be lacking.  If they show up once a week or less that becomes the norm.  They fail to understand how much a visit or phone call means to those that are being taken care of.  It also helps the caregiver in that they don't have to make excuses for why family doesn't call or show up on a regular basis. They shouldn't have to call them to ask them to stop by or at least make a phone call on a regular basis.

For those being taken care of they often feel that they are no longer of importance, forgotten or have been written off because they are of no use anymore.

They want to know what is going on in their children or grandchildren's lives and friends.

I have found this to be true after speaking with other caregivers that I have met over the years.

<u>Do You Own Your Own Home or Are You Leasing One?</u>

Your home is it possible for you to financially maintain It for a long period of time if necessary?  It is important to be able to maintain your own space if at all possible.  Even an hour of respite to your "own" space is of value to you in being able to deal with all that is now on your "shoulders".

## Are You Willing to Give Up Your Career?

Can you take time away from your work?  Have you worked a long time to reach a certain status within your field?  How is that status going to be affected if you are away from it for a long period of time?

Working part time or the ability now to be able to work on the internet on-line are viable options.  Not only creating income but keeping you up to date in the business world

## Are You Willing Move Into Their Home or They Move In With You?

Either way it will totally disrupt your life.  Your lifestyle and theirs are most likely different.  This can cause conflicts which have nothing to do with them being right or wrong.   It is basically a generation gap.  When taking care of a family member you need to be flexible in order for it to work.


## Is Alzheimer's Involved?

There is no easy answer for taking care of an Alzheimer's patient, what works today, will not tomorrow. There are so many phases of this disease it is a journey that you have to handle one day at a time.

Are you prepared to have someone not know who you are?  Are they quiet or combative?  This can sometimes depend on the relationship you have had thru-out your life with them.   Do they wander or stay within the confines of their home?  There now is an abundance of information available to help someone understand the disease, which was not readily available when I dealt with it.

It is absolutely necessary to find out all that you can about Alzheimer's and to have it diagnosed as opposed to age related dementia.  There are distinct differences with Alzheimer's disease.

## Do You Have Patience?

You need the ability to adapt to their way of life.  The way you do things and how they do them are probably totally different, which can lead to many disagreements.  What they like to eat could be entirely different from what you like.

You have to be able to adapt to any given situation. Can you deal with Doctors appointments, hospitals, and tons of paperwork?  Everything seems to be in slow motion when you are trying to resolve an issue.

Trying to get answers to questions from providers is a job in itself,  sitting in waiting rooms becomes the norm for doctor appointments, the emergency room is even worse.


## Do You Believe It Will Be Short Term, i.e. 2 years?

You have decided to take on the task of being a caregiver.  You set an amount of time that you are willing to take this on, under the auspices that arrangements such as assisted living, a nursing home, or for someone to live in if necessary can be made during this time frame.  Obviously financial considerations can play a part in these decisions and the amount of care that is needed.

Unfortunately, none of these things usually happen, by the 2$^{nd}$ year you are already too involved to walk away and the guilt starts setting in just thinking about it.

With aging people you can never know what will happen from day to day.  A fall can be disastrous, dementia, loss of sight or hearing, losing a license to drive etc. etc., the list grows on a daily basis.

## Are You Prepared to Give Up Your Social Life?

There is little of it; because of not knowing what is going to happen from day to day.  It is next to impossible to make plans and if you do the guilt factor kicks in about leaving them, even for a few hours.  Finding someone who is reliable to step in for you is easier said than done.

The longer you are a caregiver the opportunity to socialize becomes less as their needs become more involved. Most people don't want to hear about caregiving especially if they have never done it.  You have less and less in common with those you once socialized with on a regular basis. Your conversation now revolves around being a caregiver and this is not a very exciting or stimulating conversation to others, especially when you are "socializing".


## Do You Believe Your Friends Will Stick By You?

You have stuck by your friends thru thick and thin in times past, surely they will be there for you.

Unfortunately the reality is some can't understand or don't want to deal with the commitment you have made. You are basically in a 24-7 day a week job, with little if any time off.

Learning who your true friends are will likely be a surprise.  Some will disappoint you and others will surprise you.

The friends that do stay by your side will be an important part of your life, as you need someone to "vent" to as well as just be able to say or do nothing without them trying to get you to talk or go somewhere.  The main problem being is you have become isolated from those you once were surrounded by; it's a major adjustment that takes place in your life.

I like the saying "there is a time and place for everything and everyone"; it fits this time in your life.

## If You Have Savings Do You Think You Might Need Them?

Will you need to use your savings at some point, if you do this can be very stressful to you.  You don't want to disclose it to whomever you are taking care of, but you could be jeopardizing your own future needs.  The longer you are a caregiver, the more stressful it will be to maintain your own home or to just take care of yourself and your needs.

## Would You Feel Guilty Saying No?

Telling your parent or loved one you will not be able to become their caregiver could be difficult, in most cases they were there for you and it would be selfish of you to deny them. If you have any angst at all, you need to explore all options. Caregiving will change your life if it becomes long term.

You should never feel guilty about saying no.

All of the previous questions and answers were part of my caregiving experiences.  Most of the caregivers I have spoken with in the past few years have had to deal with some if not all of the above circumstances.

Every situation has its own set of circumstances that needs to have serious consideration before making a commitment.  In some cases obviously money is a problem and there is not any easy choice.  If you do have options available you should give those options a close look that relate to your own personal situation before making any decision.

Whether you are the caregiver or you have the ability to hire one, being prepared with any and all information that is available is valuable.

# MENTAL STRESSES OF WATCHING A LOVED ONE DETERIORATE

Each time you have to call 911 and sit in the ER waiting room for hours at a time not knowing if this is it, or another round of endless tests it increases the stress level.  If they are admitted for more than a few days, physical therapy more than likely will follow in order to keep them mobile. It could mean them being admitted to a facility for a given amount of time upon their discharge from the hospital, followed by a therapist coming to the home.  If they do go to rehab it is imperative that you check on them daily by phone or in person.

The less someone is able to get around and the more dependent they become on you the guiltier it makes them feel.  They feel they are of no use to anyone and that they are taking away from your life – it then prompts them into saying "I wish I were dead", "why am I still here?", " I am of no use to anyone", all my friends are gone".  All of the above sayings can escalate into them asking for a gun, pills, etc. to end it all.   This in itself can put an undue amount of stress on the caregiver.

You as the caregiver feel guilty because you are tired of all the added responsibilities to your life.  The isolation from any sense of normalcy in your life becomes more stressful the longer you are involved.

It is difficult to watch a once vibrant person slowly fail, whether it is from memory loss, eyesight, and hearing, being able to walk, or any number of other physical problems. When everyday living becomes just an existence and not much more it is depressing for the patient.  Being able to keep a positive attitude as the caregiver becomes harder and harder to maintain as you have to make decisions regarding your loved one(s) care, which could include Hospice Care.

If the person you are taking care of is mentally aware, they are more susceptible to depression as time goes on.

Each case involving Alzheimer's is different,  watching someone with the slow degradation of  the brain, robbing their ability to think, communicate ,  or recognize you is not as stressful for them as they don't understand as the disease progresses. There are some things that are typical in all Alzheimer's cases.  For the caregiver it is another added stress. The ability for you to adapt to this disease that is affecting who you are taking care of is of utmost importance. There are many sources now available for information.

I recognized the possibility of my parent having Alzheimer's disease because of being around and seeing firsthand the effects of it on a friends' Father.  The beginning stages were very familiar to me, they both had gotten lost going grocery shopping, not knowing how to get home.  They both hid food and other items thru-out their homes and became accusatory as to you having misplaced the items.  It was not unusual to find rotten food in a closet etc.  Also short term memory became more prominent.

If you think there is a possibility of someone having Alzheimer's, the sooner you have them tested the better.  Testing should be done thru a Memory Center that specializes in Alzheimer's disease.  The abundance of information now available will help you in decisions that will have to be made as to their care as the disease progresses.

# PERSONAL HYGIENE

Are you prepared to bathe your parents or loved one, to empty potty chairs and clean them, to dress them, deal with diapers in some cases?  If they have injuries from scrapes or falls, are you able to handle changing bandages if needed.

The embarrassment for them is degrading when dealing with personal care.  You more than likely could never have imagined doing many of the tasks that are needed. Unfortunately, some if not all and more will happen at some point in time.

If you are caregiving for a person with Alzheimer's, it is not uncommon for them to forget how to bathe,

brush their teeth or comb their hair
and many other personal tasks as the
disease progresses.   You have to learn
to adapt and be creative to get them
to do basic hygiene.

# FAMILY AND FRIENDS INVOLVEMENT

Caregiving almost always falls upon one person, whether you have siblings or other relatives.  They will tell you what a great job you are doing, but when you try to relate to them what is occurring with your parent(s) or loved ones they are in in many cases in complete denial.  They do not believe the situation is as difficult as you describe

When family members or friends only stop in for an hour or so once a week or less often, it is such a bright spot for them that it gives them a brief period of energy and they really don't want them to know how bad they are. With that the person visiting thinks there is no way that things could be as bad as you tell them.  They often think you are making things up in order to get attention, or their help which they truly believe is not necessary.

In some cases they can't even understand the necessity for you having to be there all the time. Knowing this in advance should be helpful in your expectations of what other family members or friend's involvement will be.  The only person who is going to really understand a caregiver is another caregiver.

Friends who remain in contact either by phone or dropping by are a bright spot for anyone that is being cared for.  Reminiscing about days past and the things they had done in their live gives them respite as to what is happening now.

For family and friends I cannot state how important a phone call or a visit is for both caregiver and the one(s) being cared for.  It helps to break up the routine for all involved.

Interacting with someone other than a doctor or nurse, or resolving problems on the phone or otherwise it gives everyone a needed break.

# MEDICAL PROFESSION

The longer the illness goes on the more involved you will be with doctors, nurses, hospitals, healthcare workers and medications.  You think you are frustrated already, well hang on to your hat!  There will be wasted hours in doctor's offices waiting for appointments that are never on time, multiple trips to the emergency room, once again waiting for them to be seen

I would tell any caregiver to purchase a "pill book".  Since the medical profession has become so specialized now, it can become a serious problem with prescription medications.  The wrong combinations can be lethal to your loved one.

If the doctor is caring and responsible, he will welcome your input and observations.   This can be invaluable information as to the overall wellbeing of your parent(s) or loved one.

Another recurring problem is submitting patients to repeated testing.   Chest x-rays, Cat Scans, MRI's seem to be high on list of being done repeatedly.   There is a need for them, but they can be overdone.  This can cause great anxiety not only for the patient, but for the caregiver as well.

Lastly, you need all the information you can get if you are the caregiver in order to give them the best care you can give at home. Persistence is key, even if you are annoying the healthcare professionals; they are being paid for their services. Being pleasant to whom you are

speaking, but make it clear you need
the information requested.  If you are
lucky their doctors will take the time
to share with you the information that
is necessary, if you have a question
ask it, there is no good reason for it
not to be answered!

# MEDICARE/SUPPLEMENTAL HEALTH INSURANCE BILLINGS

Keeping track of billings can be one of your ongoing nightmares.  If you don't keep up-to-date with it, you will spend countless hours on the phone, writing letters, etc.  Trying to find out what has or has not been billed and whether or not it has been paid.   It is also important because double billings have occurred on more than one occasion and charges have been known to appear for services that were never done.

If you don't keep up with billing statements from Medicare and your insurers, you could be subjected to threatening phone calls or letters from providers or their collection agencies.

You definitely don't need to add this aggravation to your growing list of responsibilities.   Unfortunately billing mistakes happen more often than one would think.

# DEALING WITH GOVERNMENT AGENCIES

Applying for help from government agencies can be time consuming and frustrating.   Before you even think about applying for anything make sure you take the time to put together a file with the following items:


Birth Certificate(s)

Marriage Certificate

Wills and Trust Papers

Current Banking Statements

Brokerage Statements

Stock Certificates

Insurance Policies

Tax Returns

Social Security Card(s)

Driver's License(s)

Power of Attorney (if needed)


Some or all of the above items will be requested at some point in time whether it is for hospitals, doctors, nursing homes, etc.

If you need to apply for Medicaid you will need all the above items listed and more than likely Power Of Attorney, so that you can file the application if the person be cared for is not able to file on their own.

Applying for Medicaid approval for nursing home care is a time consuming process.  Just getting the initial appointment can take several weeks.   Depending on who is handling your application it is best to be prepared for delays

It is to your benefit to find out in advance what the requirements are in your state if you ever need any of the government services.  Most of the information is readily available on the internet if you look under your state website.   Having the information readily available ahead of time could save you hours and hours of time and frustration.

# NURSING HOME/ASSISTED LIVING FACILITIES

If it comes to one of these choices, go visit them ahead of time – don't make an appointment, the whole point is to observe what is going on. Do you see people in wheelchairs sitting in the hallways?  Are the premises clean?  Is there a separate Alzheimer's care unit if necessary? What type of activities do they have available for those who can participate?

You can also go on line and find out about inspections/complaints to a particular nursing home or assisted living facility.

If you have to place someone in a home, never visit at the same time or same day if you can possibly make those arrangements.  This is the best way to find out how they are being taken care of.

If you see or are told of something wrong report it immediately to the main office and request a copy of your complaint for your own records.

Keep a record of communications with the facility no matter what the means of communication is:  by telephone, email, text or whatever communication you use.  Note what the conversation was in regards to and who you spoke with or contacted.

Hopefully you never need to use any of this information, but there are circumstances where it could be important to have.

# EPILOGUE

In conclusion, it is my hope that this will help someone to see and understand what lies ahead of them if they are to become a caregiver.  I certainly had no idea.

Being a caregiver was the hardest job I had ever undertaken in my life. Would I have changed anything? Knowing what I know now there were many things that could have been done which would have made it much easier.

The rewards are few, the losses can be great.  Caregiving is a major undertaking.  It is my hope that some or all that I have written will be of use to someone else.

I have never regretted taking care of them, it is one of life's journeys that some of us are meant to take.

I certainly learned about my own strengths and weaknesses thru-out the course of years involved in their caregiving.

The most important thing is that once it ends you will be forever changed.  You might think you can just jump back into your life.  If you have been a caregiver for several years, you will feel not only the loss of those you took care of, but your Job is over and now where do you start again.  You more than likely have been isolated to varying degrees from all that you did before you went on this journey.  It is not easy to readjust to "living" again.  Much depends on the circumstances surrounding your own caregiving experience, I still learn on a regular basis from caregivers that I meet. I highly suggest one keep a journal at the end of the day, this is a way of releasing your feelings so they don't become "bottled" up inside of you.

Two of the most important things a caregiver can have are patience and the ability to adapt to an ever-changing situation.

My hope is that what I learned as a caregiver will be of use to someone else whether they already are a caregiver or they are considering becoming one.

# "TODAY IS JUST A DAY THAT WILL BE A MEMORY TOMORROW"

**Sharon Ernst**